NEW KNOWLEDGE
INNOVATIONS
& IMPROVEMENTS

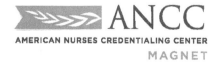

ANCC
AMERICAN NURSES CREDENTIALING CENTER
MAGNET

AMERICAN NURSES CREDENTIALING CENTER

The American Nurses Credentialing Center (ANCC) provides people and organizations in the nursing profession with the tools they need on their journey to excellence. ANCC recognizes healthcare organizations for nursing excellence through the Magnet Recognition Program®. ANCC is the largest and most prestigious nurse-credentialing organization in the United States.

Commission on Magnet® Recognition

The ANCC's Commission on Magnet® Recognition is a voluntary governing body that oversees the Magnet Recognition Program. Commission members are appointed by the ANCC's board of directors and are representatives from various sectors of the nursing community, which includes nursing executive leaders, nurse managers, staff nurses, long-term-care nurses, and advanced practice registered nurses. One commission member represents public consumers. The Commission on Magnet Recognition makes the final determination of award designation.

Magnet® Appraisers

Appraisers are leading expert nurses with demonstrated expertise and experience in various organizational and specialty backgrounds relevant to the Magnet Recognition Program. They evaluate applicant documents, conduct site visits, and prepare the final report to the Commission on Magnet Recognition. Appraisers are selected through a competitive application process. All appraisers undergo intensive training on the interpretation and evaluation of Sources of Evidence for the Magnet appraisal process before being assigned to any appraiser team.

Magnet® Program Office

The ANCC's Magnet program office staff manages and coordinates all aspects of the application and appraisal process. Contact information is available at www.nursecredentialing.org/magnet/magnetcontacts.

Published by American Nurses Credentialing Center
8515 Georgia Avenue, Suite 400
Silver Spring, MD 20910-3492

Disclaimers:

Please note: this is an abridged version of the Magnet Recognition Program Application Manual. If your organization is considering pursuing Magnet recognition, the 2019 edition of the Magnet Manual is essential for understanding the full scope of application requirements. It is the only authorized publication that provides detailed information on the instructions and process for documentation submission. To order a copy of the 2019 Magnet Manual or obtain additional information about the Magnet Recognition Program, visit our website at www.nursecredentialing.org/magnet.

The Magnet Vision

Magnet® organizations will serve as the fount of knowledge and expertise for the delivery of nursing care globally. They will be solidly grounded in core Magnet principles, flexible, and constantly striving for discovery and innovation. They will lead the reformation of health care; the discipline of nursing; and care of the patient, family, and community.

—*The Commission on Magnet Recognition, 2008*

Contents

Preface

On behalf of the American Nurses Credentialing Center (ANCC), we are pleased to present the 2019 edition of ANCC's *Magnet® Application Manual*. This valuable resource contains information and instructions to guide Magnet-recognized organizations and those considering the Journey to Magnet Excellence™.

ANCC's Magnet designation is the highest and most prestigious credential a healthcare organization can achieve for nursing excellence and quality patient care. This outcomes-driven credential brings both external prestige and wide-ranging internal benefits including improved patient outcomes, nurse satisfaction and retention, and reduced costs.

The revisions to the 2019 *Magnet® Application Manual* are rooted in a strong evidence base which spans twenty years of research and development. They create relevance for the Magnet journey by relating to the significant changes we are seeing in healthcare delivery systems around the world. The 2019 Manual clarifies previous standards, reduces the amount of information requested, and further simplifies the document submission process. Our continued focus on and strengthening of the outcomes standards will help all organizations demonstrate the value nursing brings to the patient, the organization, and the community.

Magnet designation is available to any healthcare organization regardless of size, setting, or location. Many organizations find the Journey to Magnet Excellence a valuable process to identify and improve processes, nursing structure, and ultimately deliver stronger, patient-centered outcomes.

The 2019 standards continue to raise the bar as the gold standard for nursing care delivery, new nursing knowledge, and evidence-based clinical quality in healthcare organizations around the world. The Commission on Magnet Recognition and ANCC's Magnet Recognition Program® staff trust that the 2019 *Magnet® Application Manual* will strengthen your commitment to these values and inspire you on the Journey to Magnet Excellence.

Donna S. Havens, PhD, RN, FAAN
Chair, Commission on Magnet Recognition

Jeffrey N. Doucette, DNP, RN, CENP, FACHE, NEA-BC
Vice President, Magnet Recognition Program

Chapter 1

THE MAGNET® MODEL

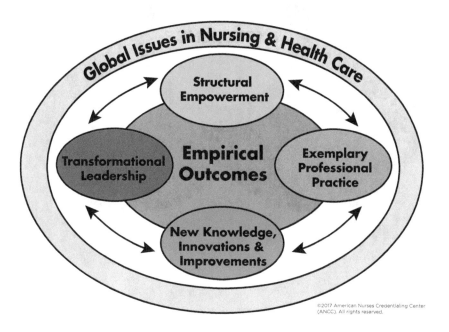

The Forces of Magnetism that were identified more than thirty years ago have remained remarkably stable—a testament to their enduring value. The Magnet Recognition Program® evolved over time in response to changes in the healthcare environment.

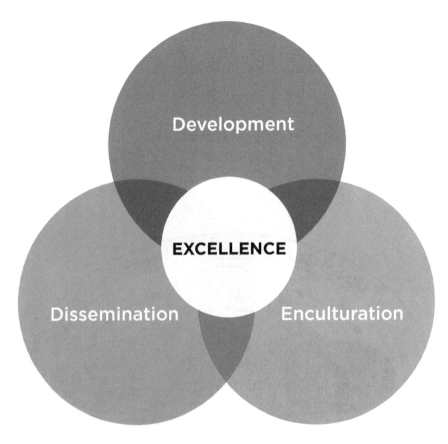

Figure 1.1. Triaxial Diagram

Statistical Foundation: The Empirical Model

In 2007, the American Nurses Credentialing Center (ANCC) commissioned a statistical analysis of final appraisal scores for applicants under the 2005 *Magnet Recognition Program Application Manual* (ANCC 2004). The project goal was to examine the relationships among the Forces of Magnetism by investigating alternative frameworks for structuring the Sources of Evidence* (SOEs)

---

* This formatting indicates that these words and phrases are defined in the Key Terms. Please refer to the Key Terms on pages 35–42 for full explanations of these terms.

and to inform development of the new Magnet Model. The newly developed Magnet Model provided a new perspective on the SOEs and how they interplay to create a work environment that supports excellence in nursing.

Through a combination of factor analysis, cluster analysis, and multidimensional scaling, the final SOEs scores were examined to determine how they might be organized based solely on their empirical properties. The results suggested an alternative framework for grouping the SOEs. The empiric model yielded from this analysis informed the conceptual development of the current Magnet Model.

Each subsequent manual has utilized a similar rigorous process, resulting in Magnet organizations creating a continued culture of excellence and innovation in nursing. Excellence is determined through the evaluation of examples demonstrating the infrastructure for excellence. The examples, provided by Magnet organizations, incorporate the structure and process used to achieve improved outcomes demonstrate how the structures and processes are present and operationalized within the organization.

Any narrative addressing SOEs must reflect compliance across the breadth and depth of the organization, wherever nursing is practiced. The Magnet program office (MPO) conducted an extensive review of final appraisal reports for written documentation that supported a site visit and incorporated the results into the 2019 Application Manual. Successful organizations demonstrated the development, dissemination, and enculturation of the Sources of Evidence.

Chapter 2

ORGANIZATIONAL OVERVIEW AND SOURCES OF EVIDENCE: NARRATIVE AND DOCUMENTATION REQUIREMENTS

Organizational Overview

The Organizational Overview requests documents and information that are foundational to Magnet® Organizations. In order for the appraisers to progress to the review of the component Sources of Evidence (SOEs), verification of all Organizational Overview items must first occur. If it is determined that any Organizational Overview items are missing, the applicant will be given the opportunity to provide the missing information one time only. If this should occur, the evaluation of the healthcare organization's documentation for Magnet designation under the Magnet Recognition Program® will be temporarily suspended and the evaluation process will not proceed until the requested information has been received. Organizations will have five business days to provide the requested information. After receipt of the organization overview items, the review will resume. When this review is concluded, the possible outcomes are a site visit, request for additional documentation, or denial.

Source of Evidence (SOE) Example Types

It is important to understand the SOE types before writing to the requirement. The SOE type will determine the format and supporting evidence required.

The 2019 Magnet® Application Manual contains two types of SOE examples:

EMPIRICAL OUTCOMES (EOS)

▸ Follow presentation guidelines found on page 11.

▸ Evidence must be presented as outcome data.

▸ All data must be within the forty-eight-month timeline.

▸ A limited number of EO sources require specific supporting documentation.

▸ Unique EO presentations are required for nurse certification, nurse education, nurse satisfaction, nurse-sensitive indicators, and patient satisfaction. Presentation requirements can be found with the corresponding SOE.

SOURCES OF EVIDENCE (SOES) NOT INCLUDING EMPIRICAL OUTCOMES (EOS)

Applicants will write narrative statements to address the SOEs. Descriptions of processes or programs must be accompanied by examples to illustrate how each is operationalized. The written document should provide examples from different departments or units to represent a variety of specialties and nursing leadership.

The applicant is required to submit a separate narrative for each SOE.

The applicant must clearly identify the SOE being addressed in each piece of the narrative.

▸ Narrative statements should be straightforward and concise and should not include extraneous information.

▸ Evidence should support and substantiate the narrative, providing verification that what is stated in the narrative actually exists in the organization.

▸ Evidence is limited to five items per SOE example.

Note: Examples of acceptable evidence include copies of policies and procedures, meeting minutes, various types of correspondence, data, rosters, and screenshots. Photographs and testimonials are not considered evidence.

Section V

NEW KNOWLEDGE, INNOVATIONS, AND IMPROVEMENTS (NK)

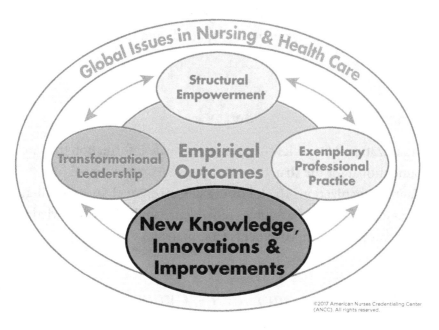

The intent of New Knowledge, Innovations, and Improvements (NK) component is to reflect:

▶ The organization supports the advancement of
nursing research[*].

---

* This formatting indicates that these words and phrases are defined in the Key Terms. Please refer to the Key Terms on pages 35–42 for full explanations of these terms.

- Nurses disseminate the organization's nursing research findings to internal and external audiences.

- Clinical nurses evaluate and use evidence-based findings in their practice.

- Innovation in nursing is supported and encouraged.

- Nurses are involved with the design and implementation of technology to enhance the patient experience and nursing practice.

- Nurses are involved in the design and implementation of work flow improvements and space design to enhance nursing practice.

Organizational Overview

Organizational Overview documents provide information that are foundational for the structures and processes enculturated in a Magnet organization. The following Organizational Overview items are associated with the Sources of Evidence in the New Knowledge, Innovations, and Improvements Component.

NEW KNOWLEDGE, INNOVATIONS, AND IMPROVEMENTS (NK)

9. Provide the policies, procedures, charters, attestation, or bylaws (including institutional review board) that:

   - Protect the rights of participants in human subject research.

   - Designates at least one nurse must be a voting member of the governing body responsible for the protection of human research participants.

OR

Provide a letter signed and dated by the chair of the governing body responsible for the protection of human research participants that attests to this requirement.

▸ If providing an attestation of "at least one nurse is a voting member on the governing body," the template provided on the website is required. http://www.nursecredentialing.org/ Magnet/Magnet-FormsTemplates/Magnet-TablesTemplates/ ResearchTable.

Note: Membership of at least one nurse as a voting member of the governing body must include the timeframe of all studies, presented on the research table (see OO10).

10. Provide table of nursing research studies (ongoing and completed) within the most recent forty-eight months.

▸ Required table can be found at http://www. nursecredentialing.org/Magnet/Magnet-FormsTemplates/ Magnet-TablesTemplates/ResearchTable.

Empirical Outcomes

Throughout this application manual, in each of the model components, the EOs are requested as SOEs.

For all New Knowledge, Innovations, and Improvements Outcomes presentations, follow the directions below.

When responding to an EO, both the goal statement and the supporting evidence must address an outcome measure. The data is best presented as a ratio (e.g., rates, percentiles, percentages). There are limited exceptions for raw data, such as sentinel event data.

Narratives must be presented using the following format:

Problem

▸ Describe the problem that you worked to improve

▸ Describe the pre-intervention outcome data that drove the goal and initiative (must have occurred within the forty-eight months prior to documentation submission)

Goal statement

▸ State the goal(s) that is the desired improvement.

▸ Identify the outcome measure that aligns with the goal to demonstrate the improvement(s) (e.g., errors, incidents, satisfaction, clinical indicator).

▸ Include the location of the desired improvement.

Participants

▸ List participants involved in the planning and intervention or initiative. Include name, discipline, title, and department.

Description of the intervention

▸ Activities that took place to facilitate change or improvement (include the dates of the work).

▸ Describe the action(s) that had an impact on the problem and resulted in the achievement of the outcome.

- Include where the intervention(s) occurred (e.g., unit, department, product line, organization).

- Include the timeline of date(s) when the intervention(s) or initiative(s) took place.

- The pre-intervention data and interventions) must have occurred within the forty-eight months prior to documentation submission.

Outcome

- For Magnet purposes, an outcome is quantitative evidence related to the impact of structure and process (intervention) on the patient, nursing workforce, organization, and consumer. These outcomes are dynamic and measurable.

- **Trended data** (minimum of one pre-intervention data point and three post-intervention data points) demonstrating an improved trend.

- Pre-intervention data and post-intervention data must be displayed to indicate the effect of an intervention.

- The trended data must be displayed as a graph and table with data elements clearly provided.

Data display requirements

- The graph must include dates, times, location of intervention and title.

- A legend must be included.

- Indicate on the graph the date(s) for pre-intervention data, intervention(s) or initiative(s), and post-intervention data.

- The x-axis units-of-time must be the same for pre-intervention, intervention, and post-intervention data (e.g., quarters, months).

- The y-axis units of measure represent the desired outcome. Data must be presented as ratio (e.g., rates, percentiles, percentages). Additionally, the unit of measure (e.g., percent to percent, whole number to whole number) must be consistent throughout the data collection period.

- If data are presented for a fiscal year, the period of time defining the fiscal year must be defined with calendar year equivalent (January to December and year; June to May and year).

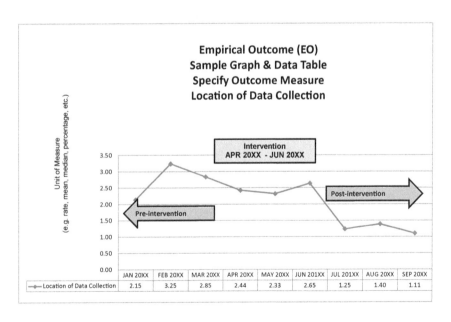

Figure V.1 Empirical Outcomes (EO) Sample Graph and Data Table

Source of Evidence (excluding Empirical Outcomes)

▹ Each key element within the SOE must be described and supported with evidence.

▹ Limit evidence to no more than five items per SOE example.

▹ Ensure all protected health information (PHI) has been redacted.

Note:

▸ All organizations with **ambulatory care setting(s)** are required to provide a minimum of one ambulatory care example for NK6EO and NK7EO

▸ Data for all EO ambulatory examples must provide description of work done and outcome data, specific to the provided ambulatory setting.

RESEARCH

NK1:

Provide a synopsis of one completed institutional review board-approved (IRB-approved) nursing research study.

Note: The nursing research study must have been conducted within the applicant organization.

Use format provided below.

Study overview

▸ Title of Study

▸ IRB approval date and type of review (i.e., full board, expedited, exempt)

▸ Study start date

▸ Study completed date

Note: For Magnet purposes, "completed study" refers to a study that has concluded to the point of analysis and from which initial implications of the findings have been determined and dissemination has occurred or will occur. The study completion date must have occurred within the forty-eight months before document submission to the Magnet Recognition Program®.

Research team

▸ Nurse(s) at the organization who is (are) the principal investigator(s) (PI), co-PI, or the site PI involved in the conduct of the study.

▸ Other key personnel on research team.

Study aim(s)

▸ Study purpose, what new knowledge will be generated, or both.

Significance of the literature review (two pages maximum)

▸ Key references to support the significance.

▸ Why the study is important to nursing (e.g., the patient experience of care, patient or health outcomes, cost of care, nursing practice).

▸ What is currently known about the topic; if an intervention study, what evidence supports the intervention or innovation.

▸ Summarize the gap in current knowledge about the topic being addressed by the study.

Innovation

▸ How the study will produce actionable information for nursing.

Study design

▸ Describe the study design: Qualitative, quantitative (descriptive, correlational, quasi-experimental, experimental, or other).

▸ Research question(s), hypothesis, or both.

Sample description

▸ Type of sample (e.g., convenience, cohort, random)

▸ Inclusion and exclusion criteria

▸ Sample size

Location of study (within the applicant organization)

▸ Hospital, unit(s), ambulatory care area(s) that apply

Study procedures

▸ Procedures from initial screening through end of contact with subjects

▸ Data collection methods

Results

▸ Results of data analysis (description of sample characteristics and analysis for research questions or hypotheses)

Discussion

▸ Discussion and interpretation of the findings

▸ Implications of the findings and recommendations to the organization

NK2:

a. Provide one example, with supporting evidence, of how clinical nurses disseminated the organization's completed nursing research study to *internal* audiences.

Note:
▸ Internal audience includes individuals employed by the applicant organization.
▸ Must be a different study than presented in NK1.

AND

b. Provide one example with supporting evidence, of how clinical nurses disseminated the organization's completed nursing research study to *external* audiences.

Note
▸ External audience includes individual(s) outside of the applicant organization.
▸ Must be a different study than presented in NK1.

EVIDENCE-BASED PRACTICE

NK3:

a. Provide one example, with supporting evidence, of clinical nurses' implementation of an evidence-based practice that is new to the organization.

AND

b. Provide one example, with supporting evidence, of clinical nurses' use of evidence-based practice to revise an existing practice within the organization.

NK4:

a. Provide one example, with supporting evidence, of how clinical nurses incorporate professional specialty standards or guidelines to implement a practice new to the organization.

INNOVATION

NK5:

a. Provide one example, with supporting evidence, of an innovation within the organization involving nursing.

NK6EO:

Two examples are required (**one example *must* be from ambulatory care setting, if applicable**):

a. Provide two examples, with supporting evidence, of an improved outcome in a care setting associated with a clinical nurse(s) involvement in the adoption of technology.

▸ Outcome data must be submitted in the form of a graph with a data table.

NK7EO:

Two examples are required (**one example *must* be from ambulatory care setting, if applicable**):

a. Provide one example, with supporting evidence, of an improved outcome associated with nurse involvement with the design or redesign of work environment.

▸ Outcome data must be submitted in the form of a graph with a data table.

AND

20 | NEW KNOWLEDGE INNOVATIONS & IMPROVEMENTS

b. Provide one example, with supporting evidence, of an improved outcome associated with, clinical nurse involvement with the design or redesign of work flow in an ambulatory setting.

  ▶ Outcome data must be submitted in the form of a graph and data table.

Compliance with Local, State, and Federal Laws and Regulations

CONFIDENTIAL INFORMATION

In accordance with the Health Insurance Portability and Accountability Act (HIPAA) and other laws and regulations, inclusion of patient-specific information and employee-specific information as exhibits must be avoided. The original document should then be available for review during the site visit. Where state law prohibits review of a document, it would be exempt from display in the organization.

Applicant entities must comply with all local, state, and federal laws and regulations administered by the Occupational Safety and Health Review Commission; the Equal Employment Opportunity Commission; the US Department of Health and Human Services and other agencies that administer healthcare programs; and the US Department of Labor, the National Labor Relations Board (NLRB), or other agencies as they relate to registered nurses in the workplace. Conduct by an applicant or a Magnet®-recognized organization that results in an adverse decision by the NLRB on an unfair labor practice complaint (adoption or modification of a decision rendered by an administrative law judge); a trial court decision on a complaint of employment discrimination; a decision by the Occupational Safety and Health Administration (OSHA) regarding violations of health and safety requirements; or the suspension or exclusion of a hospital from participation in a federal healthcare program will warrant review and action by the Commission on Magnet Recognition (COM).

Note: If protected health information (PHI) is found during the review process, the organization will be notified and be given a deadline to remove from all sources. The appraisers will stop the review if patient-sensitive information is identified.

All identified PHI must be removed. The appraisers will provide the Sources of Evidence (SOEs) where PHI has been identified. There may be other areas in the documentation that contain PHI and it is the responsibility of the organization to find and remove or redact this information. The organization's privacy officer must be notified if PHI is identified in the written documentation. If the revised documents are not provided within the required timeline, the review is concluded.

Applicant and Magnet-recognized healthcare organizations are required to disclose, within seven business days after receipt of such a decision, all decisions by an agency or court of law that occurred within the year before application or at any time after an application is submitted. Failure of an applicant or Magnet-recognized healthcare organizations to report an adverse decision by the NLRB on an unfair labor practice complaint (adoption or modification of a decision rendered by an administrative law judge); a trial court decision on a complaint of employment discrimination; a decision by OSHA regarding violations of health and safety requirements; or the suspension or exclusion of a hospital from participation in a federal healthcare program may result in denial of a pending application for initial designation or redesignation, revocation of recognition, or other adverse action.

Organizations that have their Magnet designation revoked or are prevented from continuing the application process because of an adverse decision are prohibited from reapplying for Magnet designation for a period of one year after the adverse decision.

Preparation of Written Documentation

The required contents submitted for review contributes information critical to the appraisal process. This content includes:

▸ Demographic report submitted via the DDCT portal

▸ Organizational overview

▸ SOEs

Timeline:

▸ All narrative and evidence must occur within the forty-eight months prior to document submission. This includes narratives, data, and supporting evidence and exhibits.

▸ Nurse satisfaction must be within thirty months prior to document submission.

▸ Nurse-sensitive indicators (inpatient and ambulatory) and patient satisfaction (inpatient and ambulatory) must be the most recent eight quarters.

The SOEs statements in the 2019 Magnet® Application Manual depict requirements that are present and fully operational in Magnet-recognized healthcare organizations. The term Source of Evidence should not be confused with the reference to "evidence" that is required substantiating the narrative for the example.

Appendix A

MAGNET RECOGNITION PROGRAM® RESOURCES

Magnet Recognition Program Staff

SENIOR MAGNET® PROGRAM ANALYSTS (SMPA)

Nurses who provide independent content expertise and analysis for the Magnet Recognition Program, working with applicants, commissioners, appraisers, Magnet organizations, Magnet Program staff, and American Nurses Credentialing Center (ANCC) staff. They interface with Magnet appraisers to coordinate and manage the appraisal process and with representatives of the international community to provide guidance and interpretative analysis related to eligibility and requirements for Magnet Recognition®.

SENIOR MAGNET PROGRAM OUTCOMES ANALYST

Senior Magnet program outcomes analyst provides operational support and coordination to organizations between Magnet designations. Oversees the Demographic Data Collection Tool™ (DDCT), a web-based portal for managing compilation of required demographic data into a report. Interfaces with staff of Magnet-recognized organizations and those seeking the Magnet credential.

MAGNET PROGRAM SPECIALISTS (MPS)

Magnet program specialists (MPS) provide logistical support for the Magnet Recognition Program. Coordinate and monitor the activities of applicant and Magnet-recognized organizations throughout the various stages of the Magnet application process. Specialists interface with senior Magnet program analysts on a routine basis to ensure excellence and quality service throughout the Magnet application process.

SENIOR OPERATIONS SPECIALIST

Senior operations specialist provides operational and logistical support to the Magnet Program Staff with a variety of Magnet programs and presentations. Assists with conducting ongoing evaluation of Magnet Recognition Program processes for the Commission on Magnet Recognition(COM), appraiser pool, staff, and Magnet Recognition Program to ensure efficiency, effectiveness, and excellent customer service.

MAGNET RECOGNITION PROGRAM LEADERSHIP

Vice President, Magnet Recognition Program and Pathway to Excellence®

Director, Magnet Recognition Program

Senior Manager, Operations Magnet Recognition Program

Senior Manager, Magnet Appraiser Program

The Magnet Recognition Program Website

http://nursecredentialing.org/Magnet:

- Application

- Manual updates

- Frequently asked questions (FAQs)

- Forms and Templates (for example, unit-level crosswalk, nurse leader and **nurse manager** tables, nursing research table, template for internal review board attestation)

MAGNET LEARNING COMMUNITIES® (MLC) SUBSCRIPTION

- Two free memberships are provided with designation

- Applicants and those on the journey may purchase a membership; fees for subscription are located on our website: http://www.nursecredentialing.org/Magnet/Magnet-Learning/About.

The MLC provides the following:

- Discussion Forums: The forums include moderated discussions that bring together nurse leaders who share knowledge and experiences related to leadership, engagement, evidence-based practice, research, innovation, and outcomes.

- Education: Resources available on demand in the MLC, including the "Getting Started" webinar (provides an overview of resources, definitions, and formatting), educational vignettes (webinars lasting less than ten minutes), and more!

Critical Information Webinar

This is an invitation-only webinar, limited to Magnet and applicant organizations. The invitation is sent to the applicant chief nursing officer (CNO) and Magnet program director (MPD) when the Magnet application is received by the Magnet Program Office (MPO). Check with your assigned SMPA or MPS for registration.

In Pursuit of Excellence: Magnet Recognition Program® Guidance

This interactive work session is provided to expand the understanding of the requirements in the Magnet Application Manual. Required key elements of the organizational overview and Sources of Evidence (SOE) examples, as well as expectations for Empirical Outcome (EO) SOE data presentation, are reviewed in depth. Senior analysts present sample SOE examples, facilitate group discussion, and provide one-on-one assistance to enhance the attendees' understanding of SOEs while developing skills to successfully write to the Magnet requirements.

The class is limited to CNOs, MPDs, and key stakeholders from Magnetrecognized and Magnet applicant organizations.

Annual ANCC National Magnet Conference®

PRECONFERENCE

▷ In Pursuit of Excellence: Magnet Recognition Program Guidance

- Annual MPD session:

  - For MPDs of Magnet-recognized and Magnet applicant organizations.

DURING THE CONFERENCE

- Concurrent sessions are offered by the senior magnet program analysts.

- In addition, the senior Magnet program analysts are available for questions at the Magnet Recognition Program booth throughout the conference.

Appendix B

KEY FACTORS TO CONSIDER WHEN ADDRESSING ORGANIZATIONAL OVERVIEW ITEMS OO9, OO10, NK1, NK2A, AND NK2B

OO9. The organization's policies, procedures, charters, or bylaws designating that at least one nurse must be a voting member of the governing body responsible for the protection of human research participants, and that at least one nurse votes on nursing-related protocols.

  ▹ It is acceptable to have an outsourced IRB as long as at least one registered nurse is a voting member of that IRB. The nurse does not need to be an employee of the applicant organization.

  ▹ If a system uses one IRB, one registered nurse may represent the entire System as a voting member on that IRB.

  ▹ If more than one IRB is involved—each IRB that considers nursing-related protocols must have a registered nurse as a voting member.

OO10. A table of ongoing or completed nursing research studies within the past forty-eight months.

▶ Only nursing research studies are to be listed on the table.

▶▶ Include full IRB review, exempt, and expedited nursing research that is ongoing and/or completed in the applicant organization(s).

▶▶ Evidence-based projects and quality improvement projects should not be included on the nursing research table.

▶▶ This table includes nursing research studies that are completed or ongoing within the forty-eight months before documentation submission.

Research Matrix	Organization Initiated Nursing Research	System Initiated Nursing Research	Multi-Site Nursing Research
Individual Organization Application	PI or co-PI must be RN employed by the organization	PI or co-PI must be RN employed within the system	PI, co-PI, or site PI must be RN employed by the organization.
		If the PI or co-PI is not a staff member at the applicant organization then an RN, co-PI, or RN site PI must be employed in the applicant organization	
	Implications of the research on the applicant organization must be addressed in the research study chosen for NK1	Implications of the research on the applicant organization must be addressed in the research study chosen for NK1	Implications of the research on the applicant organization must be addressed in the research study chosen for NK1

Research Matrix	Organization Initiated Nursing Research	System Initiated Nursing Research	Multi-Site Nursing Research
System Application Each entity within the system must provide a completed nursing research table.	PI or co-PI must be RN employed by the entity within the system	PI or co-PI must be RN employed within the system	PI, co-PI, or site PI must be RN employed within the system
		RN co-PI or RN site PI must be employed at each participating entity within the system	RN co-PI or RN site PI must be employed at each participating entity within the system
	Implications of the research on the entity must be addressed in the research study chosen for NK1EO	Implications of the research on each entity within the system must be addressed in the research study chosen for NK1EO	Implications of the research on each entity within the system must be addressed in the research study chosen for NK1EO

Key Terms

For full glossary of terms see 2019 Magnet Application Manual Glossary

ambulatory care setting

"Ambulatory care nursing occurs across the continuum of care in a variety of settings, which include but are not limited to hospital-based clinic/centers, solo or group medical practices, ambulatory surgery, and diagnostic procedure centers, telehealth service environments, university and community hospital clinics, military and veterans administration settings, nurse-managed clinics, managed care organizations, colleges and educational institutions, free standing community facilities, care coordination organizations, and patient homes" (American Academy of Ambulatory Care Nursing 2011, 4). For Magnet® purposes, ambulatory care settings include emergency departments and emergency care.

certification

"A process by which a state regulatory body or nongovernmental agency or association certifies that an individual licensed to practice a profession has met certain predetermined standards specified by that profession for specialty practice. Its purpose is to assure various publics that an individual has mastered a body of knowledge and acquired skills in a particular specialty" (American Nurses Association 1979, 67).

change

"To undergo transformation, transition, or substitution: winter changed to spring" (Merriam-Webster 2014).

clinical nurse

The registered nurse who spends the majority (≥51%) of his or her time providing direct patient care.

complaint

A written statement expressing dissatisfaction with, for example, service, practice, or professionalism. In contrast, a grievance is a formal complaint filed for resolution with a grievance system or process.

enculturation

"The process by which an individual learns the traditional content of a culture and assimilates its practices and values" (Merriam-Webster 2014). This includes the process by which the values of Magnet® are disseminated throughout the depth and breadth of a healthcare organization.

error

"The failure of a planned action to be completed as intended" (an error of execution) "or the use of a wrong plan to achieve an aim" (an error of planning)" (Institute of Medicine 2000, 4). It also includes "failure of an unplanned action that should have been completed (omission)" (Institute of Medicine 2004, 330).

evidence-based practice

"A problem-solving approach to clinical decision making within a health-care organization that integrates the best available scientific evidence with the best available experiential (patient and practitioner) evidence. EBP [evidence-based practice] considers internal and external influences on practice and encourages critical thinking in the judicious application of evidence to care of the individual patient, patient population, or system" (Newhouse et al. 2005, 3–4).

implementation

"The processes involved and occurring between the decision to adopt the QI [quality improvement] innovation and the routine use of the QI innovation, or the integration of a new idea or practice into the operating system of the organization" (Burns et al. 2012, 469).

innovation

"Innovation is the application of creativity or problem solving that results in a widely adopted strategy, product, or service that meets a need in a new and different way. Innovations are about improvement in quality, cost effectiveness, or efficiency" (Kaya et al 2015, 1674).

institutional review board (IRB)

"Board of experts that must be established at each institution involved in a research process to oversee the ethical conduct of research" (DePoy and Gitlin 2016, 376). For Magnet® purposes, an organization's IRB may be internal, external, or centralized at the system level.

National Labor Relations Board (NLRB)

"Independent agency created by Congress that oversees relations between unions and employers. The board has the power to settle labor disputes and to enforce its judgments in the federal courts" (Friedman 2012).

nurse managers

Registered nurses with the accountability and supervision of all registered nurses and other healthcare providers who deliver nursing care in an inpatient or ambulatory care setting. The nurse manager is typically responsible for recruitment and retention, performance review, and professional development; is involved in the budget formulation process and quality outcomes; and helps plan for, organize, and lead the delivery of nursing care for a designated patient care area.

nurse (RN) satisfaction

For Magnet® purposes, RN satisfaction is "expressed by nurses working in … [healthcare] settings as determined by scaled responses to a uniform series of questions designed to elicit nursing staff attitudes toward specific aspects of their employment situation" (American Nurses Association 1996).

The title 'nurse manager' reflects the function of the role for the purpose of documentation submission. It is understood that registered nurses who function in a nurse manager role in the organization may not be assigned the title nurse manager.

nursing research

"Nursing research provides the scientific basis for the practice of the profession. Using multiple philosophical and theory-based approaches as well as diverse methodologies, nursing research focuses on "understanding the symptoms of illness; preventing and slowing disease or disability; finding effective approaches to achieving optimal health; and improving clinical settings where care is provided (American Association of Colleges of Nursing 2006, 1). For Magnet® purposes, nursing research may encompass studies of work environment, professional development, organizational supports, and other factors that influence nurse and nursing outcomes.

organization

A stand-alone structure or an entity; the terms can be used interchangeably where appropriate or necessary.

outcome

Quantitative and qualitative evidence related to the impact of structure and process on the patient, nursing workforce, organization, and consumer. "These outcomes are dynamic and measurable and may be reported at an individual unit, department, population, or organizational level" (Malloch and Porter-O'Grady 2010, 267). Donabedian defined outcomes as the "changes (desirable or undesirable) in individuals and populations that can be attributed to health care" (Donabedian 2003, p 46). For Magnet® purposes an outcome is quantitative evidence related to the impact of structure and process (intervention) on the patient, nursing workforce, organization, and consumer. These outcomes are dynamic and measurable.

patient

A healthcare consumer across the variety of settings; he or she might variously be called a patient, client, or resident.

patient safety

"Freedom from accidental injury; ensuring patient safety involves the establishment of operational systems and processes that minimize the likelihood of errors and maximizes the likelihood of intercepting them when they occur" (Institute of Medicine 2000, 211).

patient satisfaction

For Magnet® purposes, "patient opinion of the care received during the hospital stay [or in ambulatory/outpatient services] as determined by scaled responses to a uniform series of questions designed to elicit patient views about global aspects of care" (American Nurses Association 1996).

process

The actions involving the delivery of nursing and healthcare services to patients, including practices that are safe and ethical, autonomous, evidence-based, and focused on quality improvement. Donabedian defined process as the activities constituting health care, "including diagnosis, treatment, rehabilitation, prevention, and patient education—usually carried out by professional personnel, but also including other contributions to care, particularly by patients and their families" (Donabedian 2003, 46).

registered nurse (RN)

A nurse in the United States who holds state board licensure as a registered nurse or any new graduate or foreign nurse graduate who is awaiting state board examination results and is employed by a healthcare organization with responsibilities of an RN. In other countries, this individual will have registered with the appropriate regulatory body.

research

"Systematic inquiry that uses disciplined methods to answer questions or solve problems. The ultimate goal of research is to develop, refine, and expand knowledge" (Polit and Beck 2012, 3).

safety

One of nine optional Magnet® categories for patient satisfaction benchmarking (EP20EO and EP21EO). See also patient safety.

sentinel event

"A patient safety event (not primarily related to the natural course of the patient's illness or underlying condition) that reaches a patient and results in any of the following: death; permanent harm; severe temporary harm" (The Joint Commission 2017, PS-3).

Source of Evidence (SOE)

A statement that describes key elements required to be present and fully operational in a healthcare organization in order to achieve Magnet Recognition®. Sources of Evidence are criteria statements that identify objective indicants of how well the expectations for a Magnet® environment have been met. Source of Evidence statements are distinct from the supporting evidence that may be requested to accompany narratives addressing specific SOEs. See also supporting evidence.

standard

A criterion that expresses an agreed-upon level of performance that has been developed to characterize, measure, and provide guidance for achieving excellence in practice.

structure

The characteristics of the organization and the healthcare system, including leadership, availability of resources, and professional practice models. Donabedian defined structure as the conditions under which care is provided, including material resources, human resources, and organizational characteristics "such as the organization of the medical and nursing staffs, the presence of teaching and research functions, kinds of supervision and performance review, and methods of paying for care" (Donabedian 2003, 46).

supporting evidence

Auxiliary documentation provided to support and substantiate narratives to address Magnet® SOE criteria statements. Supporting evidence is required for selected SOEs to provide verification that what is stated in the narrative actually exists in the organization. Acceptable evidence includes, but is not limited to, copies of policies and procedures, meeting minutes, various types of correspondence, data, rosters, and screenshots. Testimonial statements and examples are not acceptable as supporting evidence. See also Source of Evidence (SOE).

technology

"The practical application of knowledge especially in a given area; a manner of accomplishing a task especially using technical processes, methods, or knowledge (Merriam-Webster 2014).

trended data

Refers to data depicting a trend, defined as "the general movement over time of a statistically detectable change; also, a statistical curve

reflecting such a change" (Merriam-Webster 2014). For Magnet®
purposes, presentations of trended data to address Empirical
Outcomes SOEs must include a minimum of one pre-intervention
data point and three post-intervention data points, all occurring
within the forty-eight months prior to documentation submission.

work flow

"The set of tasks—grouped chronologically into processes—and the
set of people or resources needed for those tasks, that are necessary to accomplish a given goal. An organization's workflow is
comprised of the set of processes it needs to accomplish, the set of
people or other resources available to perform those processes, and
the interactions among them" (Cain and Hague 2008, 1).

References

Agency for Healthcare Research and Quality. 2015. "Strategies for Improving Patient Experience: Service Recovery Programs." In *The CAHPS Ambulatory Care Improvement Guide: Practical Strategies for Improving Patient Experience* (section 6). Rockville, MD: Author. Retrieved from https://www.ahrq.gov/cahps/quality-improvement/improvement-guide/improvement-guide.html.

American Academy of Ambulatory Care Nursing. 2011. *What Is Ambulatory Care Nursing?* Retrieved from https://www.aaacn.org/what-ambulatory-care-nursing.

American Association of Colleges of Nursing. 2006. *AACN Position Statement on Nursing Research*. Washington, DC: Author. Retrieved from http://www.aacn.nche.edu/publications/position/nursing-research.

American Congress of Obstetricians and Gynecologists. 2011. *Cultural Sensitivity and Awareness in the Delivery of Health Care* (committee opinion number 493). Washington, DC: Author. Retrieved from http://www.acog.org/Resources-and-Publications/Committee-Opinions/Committee-on-Health-Care-for-Underserved-Women/Cultural-Sensitivity-and-Awareness-in-the-Delivery-of-Health-Care.

American Hospital Association. 2017. "Fast Facts on US hospitals." Retrieved from http://www.aha.org/research/rc/stat-studies/fast-facts.shtml.

American Nurses Association. 1979. *The Study of Credentialing in Nursing: A New Approach* (vol. 1, Report of the Committee). Kansas City, MO: Author.

———. 1996. *Nursing Quality Indicators: Definitions and Implications*. Washington, DC: Author.

———. 2015a. *Code of Ethics for Nurses with Interpretive Statements*. Silver Spring, MD: Author.

———. 2015b. *Nursing: Scope and Standards of Practice* (3rd ed.). Silver Spring, MD: Author.

———. 2016. *Nursing Administration: Scope and Standards of Practice* (2nd ed.). Silver Spring, MD: Author.

American Nurses Association and National Nursing Staff Development Organization. 2010. *Nursing Professional Development: Scope and Standards of Practice*. Silver Spring, MD: Author.

American Nurses Credentialing Center. 2008. *Magnet Recognition Program®: Application Manual*. Silver Spring, MD: Author.

———. 2013. *2014 Magnet® Application Manual*. Silver Spring, MD: Author.

———. 2016. *Practice Transition Accreditation Program™: 2016 Application Manual*. Silver Spring, MD: Author.

Anthony, M. K. 2006. "Professional Practice and Career Development." In D.L. Huber (ed.), *Leadership and nursing care management* (3rd ed.), 61–81. Philadelphia, PA: Saunders Elsevier.

Bass, B. M., and R. E. Riggio. 2006. *Transformational Leadership* (2nd ed.). Mahwah, NJ: Lawrence Erlbaum Associates, Inc.

Benner, P., C. Tanner, and C. Chesla. 2009. *Expertise in Nursing Practice: Caring, Clinical Judgment, and Ethics* (2nd ed). New York: Springer Publishing.

Burns, L. R., E. H. Bradley, and B. L. Weiner. 2012. *Shortell and Kaluzny's Health Care Management: Organization, Design, and Behavior* (6th ed.). Clifton Park, NY: Delmar Cengage Learning.

Cain, C., and S. Haque. 2008. "Organizational Workflow and its Impact on Work Quality." In R.G. Hughes (ed.), *Patient Safety and Quality: An Evidence-Based Handbook for Nurses* (AHRQ publication no. 08-0043). Rockville, MD: Agency for Healthcare Research and Quality. Retrieved from https://archive.ahrq.gov/professionals/clinicians-providers/resources/nursing/resources/nurseshdbk/index.html.

DePoy, E., and L. Gitlin. 2016. *Introduction to Research: Understanding and Applying Multiple Strategies* (5th ed.). St. Louis, MO: Elsevier.

Donabedian, A. 2003. *An Introduction to Quality Assurance in Health Care.* New York: Oxford University Press.

Farquharson, J. M. 2004. "Liability of the Nurse Manager." In T.D. Aiken, *Legal, Ethical, and Political Issues in Nursing* (2nd ed.), 311–36. Philadelphia, PA: F.A. Davis Company.

Friedman, J. P. (ed.). 2012. *Barron's Dictionary of Business and Economic Terms.* 5th ed. Hauppauge, NY: Barron's Educational Series, Inc.

Gardner, D. B. 2005. "Ten Lessons in Collaboration." *Online Journal of Issues in Nursing* 10 (1): 2.

Gourevitch, M. N. 2014. "Population Health and the Academic Medical Center: The Time is Right." *Academic Medicine* 89 (4): 544–49.

Griffith, J. R., and K. R. White. 2002. *The Well-Managed Healthcare Organization*, (5th ed). Chicago: Health Administration Press.

Grossman, S. C., and T. M. Valiga. 2005. *The New Leadership Challenge: Creating the Future of Nursing*, (2nd ed). Philadelphia: F.A. Davis Co.

Helmreich, R. L. 1998. "Error Management as Organisational Strategy." In *Proceedings of the IATA Human Factors Seminar* (1–7). Bangkok, Thailand, April 20–22, 1998. https://www.coursehero.com/file/6242825/10111312400/.

Institute of Medicine. 2000. *To Err is Human: Building a Safety Health System*. Washington, DC: The National Academies Press.

———. 2004. *Patient Safety: Achieving a New Standard for Care*. Washington, DC: The National Academies Press.

———. 2010. *Redesigning Continuing Education in the Health Professions*. Washington, DC: The National Academies Press.

———. 2011. *The Future of Nursing: Leading Change, Advancing Health*. Washington, DC: National Academies Press.

International Council of Nurses. 2002. "Definition of Nursing." Retrieved from http://www.icn.ch/who-we-are/icn-definition-of-nursing/.

The Joint Commission. 2017. "Patient Safety Systems (PS)." In *Comprehensive Accreditation Manual for Hospitals*, PS1–PS50. Oak Brook, IL: Joint Commission Resources. Retrieved from https://www.jointcommission.org/patient_safety_systems_chapter_for_the_hospital_program/.

Kaya, N., N. Turan, and G. O. Aydin. 2015. "A Concept Analysis of Innovation in Nursing." *Procedia—Social and Behavioral Sciences* 195: 1674–78.

Kindig, D., G. Stoddart. 2003. "What Is Population Health?" *American Journal of Public Health*, 93: 380–83.

Lake, E. T. 2002. "Development of the Practice Environment Scale of the Nursing Work Index." *Research in Nursing and Health* 25: 176–88.

Malloch, K., and T. Porter-O'Grady. 2010. *Introduction to Evidence-Based Practice in Nursing and Health Care*. Sudbury, MA: Jones and Bartlett Publishers.

Merriam-Webster. 2014. *Merriam-Webster's Collegiate Dictionary* (11th ed.). Springfield, MA: Merriam-Webster, Inc.

Mosby. 2017. *Mosby's Dictionary of Medicine, Nursing and Health Professions* (10th ed.). St. Louis, MO: Elsevier.

National Advisory Council on Nurse Education and Practice. 2013. *Achieving Health Equity through Nursing Workforce Diversity*. Retrieved from https://www.hrsa.gov/advisorycommittees/ bhpradvisory/nacnep/Reports/eleventhreport.pdf.

National Quality Forum. 2012. *Care Coordination Endorsement Maintenance 2012: Phases 1 and 2: Technical Report*. Washington, DC: Author. Retrieved from http://www.qualityforum.org/ Publications/2012/10/Care_Coordination_Phases_I_and_II__ Technical_Report.aspx.

Newhouse, R., S. Dearholt, S. Poe, L. C. Pugh, and K. White. 2005. *The Johns Hopkins Nursing Evidence-Based Practice Model*. Baltimore, MD: The Johns Hopkins Hospital and Johns Hopkins University School of Nursing.

Polit, D. F., and C. T. Beck. 2012. *Nursing Research: Generating and Assessing Evidence for Nursing Practice* (9th ed.). Philadelphia, PA: Lippincott Williams and Wilkins.

Shortell, S. M., and A. D. Kaluzny. 2006. *Health Care Management: Organization Design and Behavior* (5th ed.). Clifton Park NY: Thomson Delmar Learning.

Titzer, J. L., and M. R. Shirey. 2013. "Nurse Manager Succession Planning: A Concept Analysis." *Nursing Forum* 48 (33): 155–64.

U. S. Department of Health and Human Services Health Resources and Services Administration. 2011. *Quality Improvement: Quality Improvement Methodology Module.* Retrieved from https://www.hrsa.gov/quality/toolbox/methodology/qualityimprovement/index.html.

Vogt, W. P. 2005. *Dictionary of Statistics and Methodology: A Nontechnical Guide for the Social Sciences*, (3rd ed.). Thousand Oaks, CA: Sage Publications.

Weston, M. J. 2008. "Defining Control over Nursing Practice and Autonomy." *Journal of Nursing Administration* 38 (9): 404–8.

Witmer, A., S. D. Seifer, L. Finocchio, J. Leslie, and E. H. O'Neil. 1995. "Community Health Workers: Integral Members of the Health Care Work Force." *American Journal of Public Health* 85 (8), Pt. 1: 1055–58.

World Health Organization. 2010. *Framework for Action on Interprofessional Education and Collaborative Practice.* Geneva, Switzerland: Author. Retrieved from http://www.who.int/hrh/resources/framework_action/en/.